BODY TOXINS

How Body Toxins Can Affect Physical And Mental Health

BY PATRICIA A CARLISLE

Introduction

I want to thank you and congratulate you for choosing the book, *"BODY TOXINS: How Body Toxins Can Affect Physical And Mental Health "*.

The language surrounding what toxins are is purposely vague. The Merriam-Webster definition for toxin states, "A toxin is a poisonous substance that is a specific product of the metabolic activities of a living organism, and is usually very unstable, notably toxic when introduced into the tissues, and typically capable of inducing antibody formation."

Simply put, toxin is a harmful matter. The reason for this ambiguous language is due to the many types of toxins, all with different and potentially detrimental effects. For the purpose of clarity and consistency in our detox book, we break down toxins into three categories: Internal toxins, external toxins, and toxic behaviors.

Internal Toxins

The human body is an amazing place. It's self-defending, self-repairing, and self-poisoning. We naturally produce internal toxins simply by functioning. However, our bodies also have automatic processes in place to rid our bodies of these natural toxins and prevent build up. Our bodies are constantly burning energy in order to rebuild tissue and replace worn out, dying cells. Because of this overwhelming task, our bodies are also creating a fair amount of waste, or internal toxins, which we must break down, recycle, and eliminate.

Toxins become dangerous when it accumulates. Because our bodies are always producing toxins, they never get a break to address the toxins that have built up in the body. Instead, they're tossed to the side, where they'll sit and cause damage to surrounding organs and cells. Without help, these toxins clog your system and force your body to spend more energy to function. Things that may affect your internal toxin levels can be as basic as everyday medications. For example, proton pump inhibitors like antacids can slow digestion and lead to a reduced ability to absorb vitamins. Long-term use of Tylenol can prevent liver detoxification, and is known to be one of the leading causes of liver failure.

Signs of built up internal toxins include:

Chronic infections such as chronic sinusitis or dysbiosis of the intestinal tract. Allergic reactions, both immediate and delayed. The most common delayed sensitivities are gluten, dairy, eggs, and corn. Elevated liver enzymes.

External Toxins

If our bodies are such well-oiled machines then why are we so toxic? The simple answer is because our bodies aren't the only toxin? External toxins are the toxins outside of our bodies that an be ingested or absorbed. If you only listen to your favorite celebrity health experts, you might think toxins are only in the foods we eat. With so much focus on GMO's, and high fructose corn syrup, the everyday products filled with toxins are overlooked. External toxins can be found in everything from your daily deodorant to even your drinking water. Examples include:

Environmental Pollutants: Smoke, smog, debris, etc.

Heavy Metals Mercury: Often found in fish Lead, old paints, blinds, and canned goods.

Aluminum: Can be found in antiperspirant, deodorant, and antacids.

Mold: Can be inhaled during exposure to improperly ventilated rooms such as bathrooms or basements.

Poor Air Quality: Can be inhaled during exposure to rooms or buildings with poor ventilation or poorly maintained air filters. This can also lead to "Sick Building Syndrome," in which building occupants experience a range of symptoms from migraines to respiratory problems, but no illness can be identified. It can also be found in contaminated food and water, chemicals found in household cleaners, or pet products, Bisphenol A, and Phthalates found in soft plastics, and UV radiation.

Toxic Behaviors

As we said earlier, toxins come in a variety of shapes and sizes. While most view the toxin definition to only include physical elements, your actions and behaviors can also lead to increased toxins. For example, contact with harsh chemicals is obviously bad, but you probably don't think twice about staying late at work to finish a project. These small behaviors add up, and can lead to a significant change in your health.

Exposing yourself to stressful situation on a regular basis can be as detrimental as taking Tylenol every day. While it's normal to feel stressed every now and then, excessive stress can lead to an unhealthy diet, and overeating, mental health issues such as anxiety and depression, and lethargy.

What Is A Detox?

Now that we've covered the full toxin definition, hopefully the idea of a detox should be a little clearer. The Merriam-Webster detox definition is pretty straightforward which states: "Detox is to remove a poisonous or harmful substance." As stated earlier, your body has natural processes in place to remove waste and toxins. So, what's the point of a detox diet?

How Your Body Works

Your body has two main organs that are responsible for detoxing your entire body-the liver and the kidneys. These organs act like filters to separate the toxins from other useful nutrients.

The Liver

The liver uses a two-step process, and is your body's first wave of defense against toxins. First, enzymes transform fat-soluble toxins into an intermediate toxin. Intermediate toxins are actually more hazardous to our bodies as they're in an unstable form. Next, enzymes convert the hazardous intermediate toxin into a water-soluble toxin so that it can be pushed along and ultimately flushed out of the body.

Because the liver disposes of toxins in two sparate phases there is the potential for imbalance. To best illustrate why this can cause problems, think of your liver as a toy factory with two connected conveyor belts - the first for assembling the toys, the second for packaging the toys. If the first conveyor belt is assembling the toys faster than the second conveyor belt can package them, there's going to be trouble. In the case of your liver, instead of a build up of toys between the conveyor belts, it's the highly concentrated intermediate toxin, which can react and damage DNA.

The Kidneys & Gastrointestinal Tract

After the liver creates the new water-soluble toxin, it pushes the toxin on the kidneys and gastrointestinal tract. This is where things get complicated, so we'll revert to the previous analogy. The liver factory has packaged the toys into a form (water soluble toxin) that meets all of the requirements for the post office to ship (the right form for excretion). The post office puts the package onto a truck and sends it out on the road (the gastrointestinal tract). If everything goes smoothly, the package will be delivered and the toy is no longer the company's property (the toxin is carried out through urination).

However, if along the way, the truck encounters multiple storms (the billions of unhealthy bacteria that exist in your digestive tract) things may go wrong. The package may get damaged along the way (the ratio of healthy to unhealthy bacteria is off), and have to be returned to the factory for repackaging. This damage occurs when unhealthy bacteria transform the water-soluble toxin into a state that can be reabsorbed by your body. The toxins must then travel through the liver all over again in order to be repackaged.

Reinforcements

The body is an amazing place. When the liver and kidneys get overwhelmed, they call in for reinforcement from your backup detox organs, including your large intestine, lungs, bladder, and skin. Since detox isn't the primary function for these organs, your body must divert extra energy for them to handle the added responsibility. However, too much added work can cause stress and lead to reduced effectiveness, and allow toxins to build up over time, damaging cells and tissue. This can result in symptoms such as skin irritations, cysts, benign tumors, asthma, or arthritis.

Detox Diets

The purpose of a detox program is to support your liver and kidney functions in order to prevent an imbalance or buildup. While some workouts may boast that they'll help you "sweat out the toxins," the most effective way is to start from the inside out. Certain foods and even clays break down more effectively than others, and contain enzymes that bind to toxins and carry them through your digestive tract, easing the burden on your liver and kidneys.

Thanks again for choosing this book, I hope you enjoy it!

The trademarks that are used are without any consent, and the publication of the trademark is without permission or backing by the trademark owner. All trademarks and brands within this book are for clarifying purposes only and are the owned by the owners themselves, not affiliated with this document.

Patricia A. Carlisle, MSW, CBT

Patricia Carlisle- A Master Social Worker and a Cognitive Behavioral Therapist (CBT) gives out an expression of how important it is for an individual to take into consideration the concept of self-assessment to know what human, technical and conceptual skills they posses to perform or to achieve what they desire, or to deal with everyday life. However, every particular group of people has their own unique set of ideas, traditions and events including the frame of mind according to which people perform but there are many who faces problems and fail to maintain a healthy mind set affecting their behaviors and performance to those around them.

People like Patricia Carlisle are among those who have felt this urge of serving people and helping them out of their mental crisis towards a healthy life. She has experienced some close encounters in her personal life regarding mental health issues in her family and friends that has encouraged her to pursue this as her career.

Currently Patricia Carlisle is serving as a Certified On-Line Cognitive Behavioral Therapist with an extensive 15years of experience using Cognitive-Behavior Therapy Techniques. She envisions a world where everyone gets mental health treatment with no mental health stigma and to make it real she has already set up her own Holistic Measure Online Comprehensive Behavioral Healthcare Company after retiring from The Nord Center in The Partial Hospitalization Program (PHP) Dept for 5 years and Murtis H. Taylor Mental Health Center as a mental health counselor, psychological support technician and case manager for 10 years to emulsify her skills more professionally. Along with this, she has wrote down her passion as a clinician in 25 or more short books to help individuals and families get their life back, freeing them of the restraints of negative thinking, anxiety and depression by using different approaches. She is highly appreciated among her clients for her flexibility and professionalism of dealing with them graciously.

To reach her, make use of her direct website address: http://therapist2013.wix.com/e-therapy . As she is ready to inspire hope and contribute to health and well-being by providing the best online health care through comprehensive practice, education and research.

TABLE OF CONTENT

Chapter 1

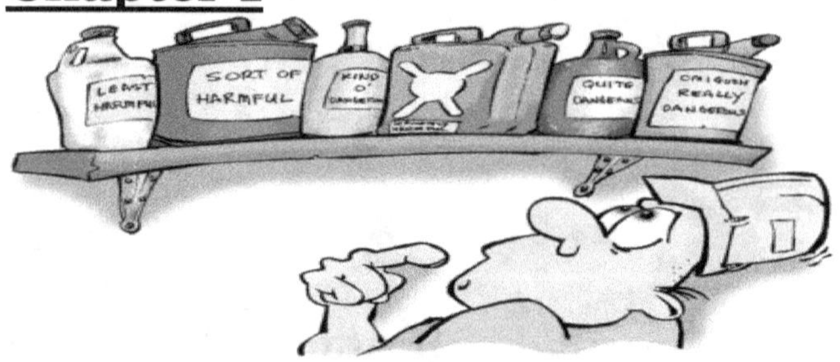

FOUR TYPES OF TOXINS HARMFUL TO OUR BODY

Our body needs to be cleansed to keep it healthy and clean. The process known as metabolism is responsible for the timely cleansing of our system. Metabolism usually takes 12 - 24 hours to complete, and at the end of the process body toxins are flushed out of the body through excretion.

If waste are not removed from the intestinal tract in time, the human anatomy has a tendency to take it back or absorb them once more in to it. They get synthesized to poisonous body toxins. The human body by nature is made to protect itself from the development of toxins to a certain extent. However, other imbalances occur to body like tiredness, nervousness etc., and simultaneously disturbs the usual functions of the body. The body toxins if remained in the body will enter other organs through circulation of blood; resulting in obesity, constipation, endocrine imbalance etc.

The four types of body toxins:

FREE RADICALS: Free radicals are the first among the body toxins which can be seen in te human body. Free radicals in correct proportion are beneficial to our system. It protects the human body from the harmful effects of chemicals and other materials. However, if they are present in the human body in excess, the outcome will be extremely harmful. Excessive free radicals produce strong corrosion and destroy body cells, augmenting chances of aging, causing different types of allergies and cardiovascular ailments.

CHOLESTEROL: Cholesterol is another toxin that can jeopardize your health. Like free radicals, cholesterol also is beneficial to the human body, if the amount is not excess. It is vital to have cholesterol in right proportion in our body to keep our organs healthy. Nevertheless, if cholesterol in take is high and continuing, the cholesterol level raises, which results in the rise of serum cholesterol, concurrently raising the risk of heart diseases. The largest part of cholesterol is created by the liver. We should be careful to keep the cholesterol level in control by avoiding high cholesterol foods.

LACTIC ACID: Lactic acid makes people exhausted. Other signs of the presence of lactic acid are hypo-dynamia, fatigue etc. Lactic acid can get build up with gluconic acid in the human body and can turn blood acidic.

URIC ACID: Uric acid is a product of metabolism. Uric acid is released by the kidneys. If the collection of uric acid is more than the usual standard, it will get collected in soft tissues, and body joints to create severe inflammation.

The toxins should be removed from our body in time, to keep our body healthy. Maintaining the stability of metabolism is the key to remove harmful toxins from our body. We should be careful to include foods that increase the metabolism rate so harmful toxins can get expelled from our system without delay and maintains the overall health of our body.

Chapter 2

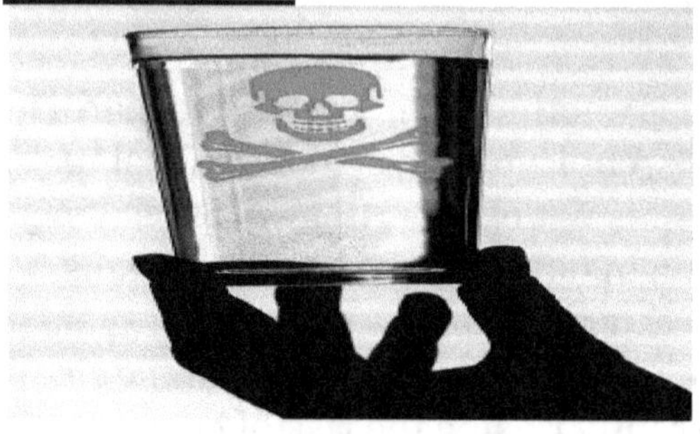

WHY YOU SHOULD DETOX YOUR BODY

According to researchers, humans themselves are the root cause for most diseases. Long working hours, stress, inappropriate nutrition, lack of sleep, smoking, and gorging on junk foods are some of the causes for change in our way of living.

Different toxins that we consume are harmful for the body in the long run, as they deteriorate the system. These toxins spread in various organs of the body gradually lead to different kinds of health problems.

Body detoxification cleanses and eradicates built up toxins and chemicals such as carbon monoxide, mercury, and lead from the system. Detoxification also helps in eradicating extra scraps presented in your body.

Things to Know About Body Detoxing

Body Detox purifies and cleanses the kidneys, lungs, colon, liver, lymph glands, and skin. It relaxes and refreshes your body from constipation, gas, acidity, skin allergies, weakness, nausea, fatigue, hair loss, and keeps you fit physically and mentally. In short, it purifies your blood and boosts blood circulation. It also helps the body to fight against diseases. Pollution is the most common problem, which affects our well-being. Even the air that you breathe is polluted.

Hence, it is important to assist your body in removing the toxins and accumulated poison from the body. Various organs of your body re□uire regular clean up and detoxification helps to do this. If your body shows any of the following signs, it is time to detox your body.

1. Fre□uent mood change

2. Gas and acidity problems

3. Tiredness or restlessness

4. Weakness or low energy level

5. Fre□uent headaches

6. Constipation

7. Digestive problems

8. Hair fall and dandruff

9. Weight gain and weight loss

10. Excessive hunger

11. Skin Infection or allergies

12. Bad breath

13. Stomach pain

14. Sluggishness

15. Depression

16. Excess or lack of sleep

17. Menstrual related problems

Similar to external cleaning, the body re□uires internal cleaning on a regular basis. You will feel good from the inside. As a result, you will be cheerful, energetic, contented, and peaceful.

Consult a health professional, if you feel you need to detoxify your body.

The following tips may help in the body detoxification process:

It is very essential that you cut down on alcohol, sugary products, inundated fats, smoking, and coffee. This is the first vital step for effective purification of the system. If you cannot control these things, the outcome will be unsatisfying. If possible, use natural and herbal products for body cleansing.

Depression and stress are also a few major hindrances in good health. They activate stress hormones into the body, thus making you feel frustrated, angry, and sad. In addition, these factors increase the toxin levels in the liver.

Remove the stressful events out of your life with a body detoxification program. Relax yourself with spiritual activities and yoga power. This will definitely make you feel better, and help you to tackle stress with positive energy.

Consume fresh fruits and leafy vegetables, which are high in fiber content. Oranges, beetroots, cabbage, radish and broccoli are good detoxifying food items. You may you can opt for herbal tea or green tea rather than consuming caffeine products.

Eat food items that have a good source of Vitamin C. This generates glutathione in the liver, which throws away harmful chemicals and toxins out from your body. One vital tip is to drink plenty of water. Indulge yourself in breathing exercises regularly for at lease 10 minutes on a daily basis.

Hydrotherapy is also a good body detox therapy, wherein you take hot a bath or shower, lie on your back for 5 minutes followed with a cold shower for 35 seconds. Next, you need to lie on the bed for about 30 minutes.

What you may not be aware of is that for optimum health, you also need to detoxify your life on mental, emotional, and spiritual levels too.

Physical toxins

Although the jury is still out on whether or not specific short-term cleanses are helpful, it is clear that your body is a master of cleansing. It must detoxify efficiently or you will get ill and eventually die.

In the days when you ate well, get plenty of exercise, clean air, and pure water to drink, our bodies will do a great job of cleansing all by themselves. If you cells don't function properly diseases such as cancer can be a result.

Mental Toxins

Your thoughts have great power to promote health or illness. Your thoughts influence brain chemistry, and the chemical messengers that go to the cells. Your thoughts can set the stage for a healing nurturing environment for your cells or a toxic environment.

Persistent negative thoughts keep you in a state of stress. This limits your body's ability to give enough energy and resources to detoxification. It also floods your body with stress hormones that need to be broken down.

A difficulty here is that not all your beliefs are conscious. Subconscious beliefs are very powerful. They are part of you and therefore your programming. Some you inherited and others you learned as a very young child. Yet they are still toxic and need to be rooted out if you want to experience good health.

Emotional Toxins

Your thoughts influence your emotional state and the two are closely linked. Thoughts fuel emotions and emotions lead to more thoughts. Eventually emotions can get "automatic". Your cells get used to the chemical that are being released and demand more from your brain.

If you want proof your emotions affect your health just notice how your body feels next time you are happy or peaceful. Notice how it feels when you are angry or upset. Occasional bursts of emotions like anger and grief can be cleansing and healthy. But when these emotions are fre□uent and out of control they become poisonous to your mind and body.

Spiritual Toxins

Unforgiveness, lack of love in all its forms, and an ungrateful spirit keep you closed off from the healing energies of your mind, body and the universe. No grudge, resentment or limiting belief is worth the amount of your natural resources and energy it uses in your mind, body and spirit. These toxic states can cause you to become ill. Sometimes negative spiritual and emotional issues are passed down from parents to children. These are toxic, low energy states. You can choose to heal them for yourself and future generations.

How To Remove Toxins From Our Body

Detox diet is a regulated diet that helps reduce the toxins in a body. Toxins could be caused by a number of substances like alcohol, tobacco, pesticides, and other elements. Detox diets help in clearing out these harmful toxins through the organs of elimination like skin, liver, kidneys etc. A detox diet strengthens the organs involved in detox and releases stored toxins. A detox program may consist of a special diet, nutritional supplements, herbs, hydrotherapy, exercise, breathing techni□ues and/or sauna.

Toxin Elimination

The most important method of removing toxins from your body is through elimination through urine and stools. It is very important to have regular bowel movements to prevent the body from developing toxic substances. Eat fibrous fruit and vegetables such as banana. You may even try flaxseed with water. This will have a mild laxative effect and help you clear your bowels. Lemon juice in water also has a slightly laxative effect and stimulates the digestive juices which are important for detox. S☐ueeze a wedge or 1/4 lemon into warm water and drink immediately after rising in the morning, and before having the flaxseed drink.

Detox diet using simple food

There are various diets available. And these need not necessarily mean fasting or eating strange and unheard of fruits or vegetables. Your diet should consist of fresh and simple fruit and vegetables that are cooked in a very simple fashion without too much spices, oils or fat, and re☐uires little preparation. Such foods are easily digestible, easily absorbed, and can be eliminated. Not only will this fresh food diet eliminate toxins, it will improve vitality and stamina, help your digestive system, you will have a better mental clarity and focus, and experience the feeling of calmness.

Chapter 3

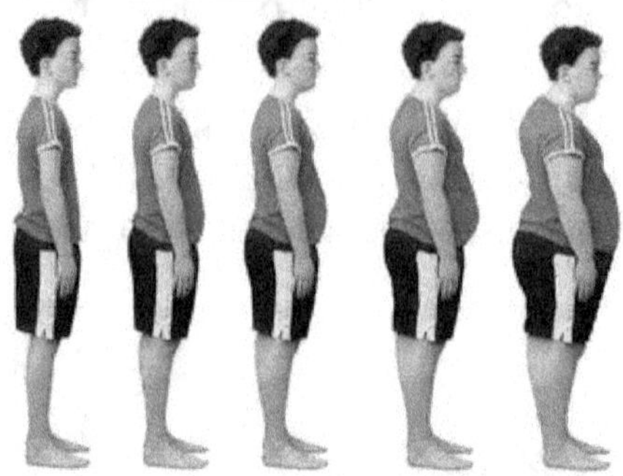

SIGNS YOUR BODY IS FULL OF TOXINS

You think you're healthy, but you don't feel vibrant. You struggle to find the energy to get through the day. You're irritable. Your stomach isn't feeling right. And all those headaches!

These types of ailments affect many of us in our daily lives. They're not serious enough to warrant a trip to the doctor or maybe you tried only to be told there was nothing wrong — but it still tend to drag you down, wearing away your resistance and leaving you feeling like you're just getting old.

I have good news for you it probably has nothing to do with aging. Instead, you may simply be surrounded by too many toxins.

Not sure? Here are seven signs to look for- and how you can clean up your system and feel better in 30 days.

1. Consistent Fatigue

Even if you're sleeping well, you may have to fight to get through the day. This could be a sign that your body is working too hard to get rid of the toxins in your body. How do you cope with fatigue? If you're answer is "more coffee" or "sweet foods," you can bet that you're only making the problem worse. That fatigue could also be in response to hormone disruptors that are zapping your immune system.

2. Weight Gain

It's never easy to lose weight, but if you're exercising daily and cutting back on calories, and you're still putting on the pounds, you could be looking at a hormonal problem. Strangely enough, our natural hormone function can be greatly affected by the toxins in our foods and personal care products. Many toxins are lipophilic, which means they are stored in body fat. These lipophilic toxins include dioxins, PCBs, and many pesticides. So it makes sense when you have an overload of these toxins it would seem impossible to lose the extra weight. You need a complete detox of your diet and personal care routine to give your body a fighting chance.

3. Bad Breath

You brush and brush, chew gum, rinse, and swallow breath mints, and still, you can't get rid of it. Bad breath is often related to digestive problems, but it can also mean that your liver is struggling to get rid of the toxins in your body. Until you tackle the problem from the source, you'll continue to scare away anyone who comes in close contact with you!

4. Constipation

The intestines get rid of a lot of toxins every day of our lives. When we're constipated, we're storing up all those toxins, allowing them to negatively affect our bodies. In addition to stomach upset, constipation can cause headaches, body aches and pains, and tiredness. It can also be related to the toxins in your life, especially if you're consuming a lot of processed foods filled with chemicals, pesticides, and preservatives.

5. Sensitivity To Scents

Strong reactions to smells — particularly fragrances — might mean that you're simply sensitive to chemicals, which many of us are. It can also mean that your body is fighting toxic overload. Particularly if you suffer headaches or stomach upset simply from scents, this may be the case.

6. Muscle Aches And Pains

If you can't tie these to your workout yesterday, could be that the toxins in your body are working away at your muscles and joints. This is more likely if you experience muscle aches on a regular basis.

7. Skin Reactions

Acne, rashes, and other skin problems may signal a toxic overload. Acne, in particular, can be related to the toxins in our diet or skin care products. Puffy eyes and eczema or psoriasis outbreaks can also be signs that you've just reached your toxic limit.

8. Fuzzy Thinking

Many toxins directly affect the brain, including aspartame and MSG (monosodium glutamate). The impact of these toxins include forgetfulness. It is important to cut out aspartame and MSG as they are excitotoxins, which means they literally excite our brain cells. Aspartame is found in many sugar-free drinks, diet foods, and toothpastes. MSG is found in many processed foods as well.

9. Unexplained Headaches

If you suffer from regular, unexplained headaches, it could be a sign that your toxic load is too high. Common toxins that cause headaches include MSG and aspartame, as discussed above. However, many other toxins also lead to headaches, including heavy metals, artificial colorings, and artificial preservatives

10. Mood Swings

If you have mood swings it can indicate that your hormones are out of balance. Some toxins, such as xenoestrogens, cause hormonal imbalances in women and men. Xenoestrogens are synthetic compounds that act like estrogen in your body. Sources include industrial compounds like PCBs, BPA, and phthalates. Avoiding plastics should have an impact on reducing your xenoestrogen load.

If your body is stressed out due to a high toxic load, your cortisol levels can get out of control. Cortisol is a hormone you release to help you deal with stress. Normal and healthy cortisol levels are highest in the morning and lowest in the evening. However, if the hormone is out of balance, in the evening its levels can be too high. This leaves you feeling really energetic and simply unable to sleep. Having insomnia can wreak havoc on your health, so it's important to get to bed on time, and to sleep at least eight hours a day.

SOLUTIONS

If you find yourself suffering from any of these ten symptoms, here are a few tips that may help:

> Support your liver with things like dandelion tea, parsley, cilantro, and milk thistle.

> Drink more water — it helps flush toxins out of your body.

> Exercise at least 30 minutes a day. Exercise gets the circulation moving, helping to move toxins along.

> Get a good daily supply of digestion-supportive probiotics, found in kefir, yogurt, sauerkraut, Kombucha tea, miso soup, tempeh, and kim chi.

> Always brush your tongue — even better, use a tongue scraper—when brushing your teeth.

> Practice deep breathing — we get rid of a lot of the toxins in our bodies through our lungs.

- ➢ Use only natural skin care products that are free of fragrances, sulfates, phthalates, parabens, and other potentially toxic ingredients, and always read labels. Use these Ingredients to avoid and have safer options.

- ➢ Choose clean, whole, and organic foods whenever possible!

Here's to living a healthy, toxin-free life!

Benefits of Body Cleansing

Body cleansing has many benefits beyond feeling great and losing weight. A proper body cleanse can give your skin a healthy glow, clear your mind, have an anti-aging effect, and help you recover your health.

Every day toxins are absorbed into our bodies including pesticides in your food, air pollution, and medications. Add to this the internal toxins created by our bodies such as those from daily metabolism and stress.

Luckily, your body has systems and organs in place to deal with these toxins. In a healthy body, toxins are dislodged, neutralized and filtered through organs like the liver or kidneys. They can then flow out of your body through your blood stream, lymphatic fluid and other daily processes.

In our industrial, modern society, we demand more of our bodies. The result is organs and a body that are overburdened and worked to the limit. You see results of this in the rise of chronic disease, auto immune diseases, and obesity when the body stores waste instead of eliminating it.

The slowing of these systems and their fluids results in kidney stones, gall stones, liver diseases, toxemia, food allergies, premature aging, and chronic disease. Here's where the benefits of body cleansing come in.

Your skin is an organ of elimination. In fact, it is your largest organ. When internal systems are slowing, your body will use this organ to try to force the toxins out. This can result in poor skin □uality including dullness and skin blemishes.

Body cleansing opens up your natural cleansing and detoxification systems. This is why one of the first noticeable benefits of cleansing is a healthy, glowing skin. As your blood stream and lymph flow easier, waste can move out through the proper internal channels.

When your blood is clearer, more oxygen and nutrients can be transported. This brings more nutrients for your body so that it can create new, fresh skin cells and collagen. This helps your skin stay toned, younger and fresh looking. More oxygen and nutrients in your blood gives your skin a healthy glow.

Fat cells act as storage for waste. If your body can not remove toxins as it should, they will be stored. This causes puffiness, weight gain and even cellulite. This can create a vicious cycle that makes it easier to gain weight, yet harder to lose it.

A body cleanse helps your body's natural cleansing systems to do what they are supposed to do - keep waste moving out. When you help this process, toxins that are stored will naturally be dislodged and removed. This is your bodies' natural survival instinct that was once suppressed because it was over burdened. Actively cleansing your body helps take the burden off.

Your body is made to kill virus, bacteria and other pathogens that can cause sickness, and even make you chronically ill. Your lymphatic system is part of your body's natural defense. It carries your white blood cells through your body. These cells attack and kill off or neutralize the "bad guys." These toxins are then sent to your lymphatic fluid so they can be transported out of your body.

When too many toxins are added to your daily dose of bacteria, virus and pathogens, your lymphatic system becomes over burdened and can become sluggish. Only so many toxins can be dealt with at a time. Your lymphatic system and organs cannot keep up so some toxins get stored.

In addition, there are some chemical toxins that your body doesn't even recognize! These are found in pesticides, tap water, air pollutants, and household cleaners. If your body doesn't recognize the toxin, it cannot kill or neutralize it, and it can easily get stored.

Chemical toxins are linked to a number of health issues including depression, auto immune disease, obesity and various cancers. Billions of pounds of harmful toxins are released into the ground, our food, water, and air. Your body needs help.

Cleansing your body helps clear toxins. This eases the burden on the lymphatic system, which frees it to do what it is meant to do; neutralize, kill and eliminate toxins. In addition, body cleansing uses natural foods and supplements that can help absorb toxins so they are more easily eliminated from your body.

As your body gets cleaner, it gets healthier. Your body's natural ability to heal itself is enhanced when the toxin load is lightened. Your lymphatic system and blood flows easier, carrying more healing oxygen and nutrients throughout your body. The results can be a stronger immunity with better health.

Chapter 4

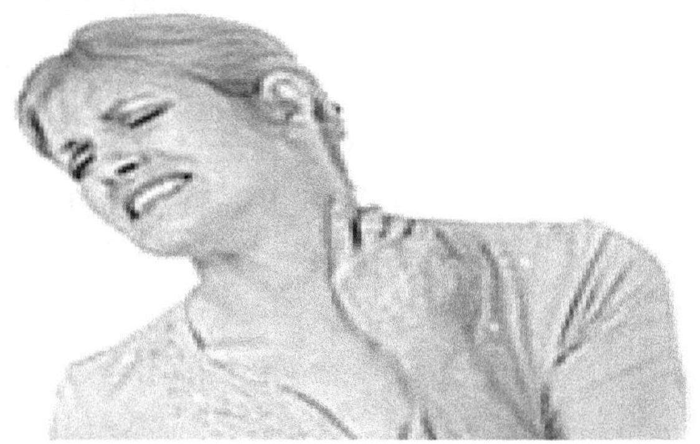

HOW TO REMOVE TOXINS FROM THE BODY

When you decide that you want to remove the toxins from your body, you will find there are innumerable methods for completing this task. The different methods for removing toxins from the body include teas, supplements, vitamins, diet, and exercise. Many different herbal teas are created specifically for detoxifying the body. When these methods are combined with a change in diet, detoxification can be completed and sustained for a healthier lifestyle.

Changing ones diet and exercise is perhaps the easiest way to remove and reduce toxins from the body. Many of the processed foods and sugars, alcohol, coffee, smoking, and other foods and drinks that a person consumes add to the toxins in their bodies. Eliminating these items from your diet and eating foods that promote circulation, and good health will begin to flush toxins from your system.

Chemicals are a big factor in the amount of toxins that are in the body. Another way to remove toxins from the body is to remove your exposure to toxins. This includes chemically based cleansers, grooming products, and other items that cause chemical reactions in the body.

One of the biggest toxin producers today that is affecting more and more people is stress. Stress releases hormones in the body that decrease the liver ability to detoxify the body. By reducing stress through proper diet and exercise, you can greatly reduce toxins in your body. Taking some yoga and meditation classes, learning relaxation techni□ues in breathing, and other stress reduction techni□ues will help you to feel better, and reduce toxins.

There are many herbs that naturally detoxify the body. These herbs are available in homeopathic remedies and teas that are available through many sources. Peppermint tea improves the circulation of blood and acts as a detoxifier. Echinacea tea forces toxins from the lymph nodes. Cilantro is a powerful detoxifer as well as garlic, and ginger root.

Among the vitamins and minerals that remove toxins is Vitamin C, B, and magnesium. Many herbal remedies that are mixed by homeopaths contain combinations of herbs, minerals, and vitamins that work together to detoxify the body.

A method for removing toxins that is growing in popularity is clay baths. Many people who go to spas include a mud bath with their massage. Calcium montmorillonite clay draws toxins out of the body as you are laying in the warm bath. It also relaxes the muscles and contains minerals and vitamins that are absorbed by the body. After getting out of the bath a lot of people notice a film on the top of the clay that are toxins floating on the surface of the bath that have been removed from the body.

Choosing which remedy, or combination of remedies to use when you are removing toxins from the body will re□uire some research and discussion with individuals who are knowledgeable in the different types of remedies, herbs, vitamins, minerals, diet, and exercise available. Finding the combination that works best for you will give you the opportunity to feel better, and enjoy a healthier lifestyle.

Chapter 5

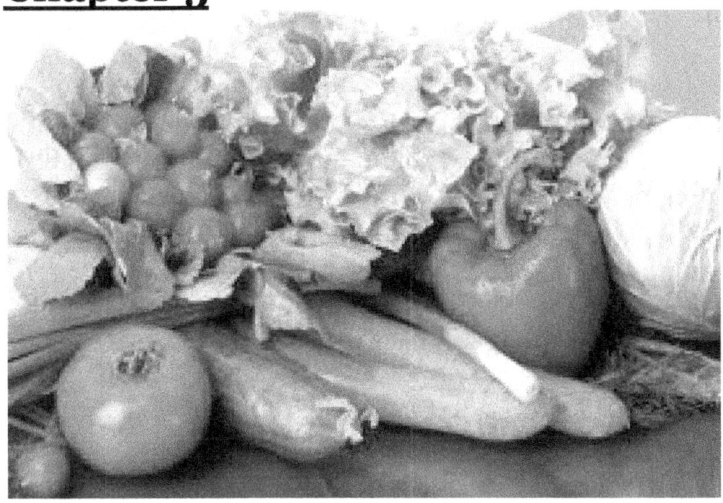

FOODS THAT REMOVE METAL TOXINS FROM THE BODY

If you are concerned about heavy metals and their effect on your health, eating certain foods may help to detoxify these toxic chemicals from your body. Heavy metals found in our teeth, our homes, and in our air can have long-lasting toxic effect on our organs, becoming lodged in the tissues of our liver, kidneys, hair, skin and bones. However, some whole foods protect our bodies from mercury, cadmium, and lead, improving our ability to eleminate them safely. Consult with your health care provider before combining natural remedies with prescription medications.

CHLORELLA: Chlorella is a green algae rich in vitamins, minerals, antioxidants and chlorophyll. In a study published in "Nutrition Research and Practice", researchers investigated the detoxifying properties of chlorella in animals given high doses of the heavy metal cadmium. Chlorella reduced the amount of cadmium that became lodged into the cellular tissues of the animals and increased the levels of cadmium that were detoxified through the urine and feces. Chlorella when taken internally can counteract the toxic and dangerous effects of heavy metals, and aid in their safe elimination from the body.

CILANTRO: Cilantro is a culinary and medicinal herb more commonly known as coriander. The leaves of the cilantro plant are rich in essential oils with anti-inflammatory, antimicrobial and detoxifying properties. According to Kevin Gianni, author of "High Raw," cilantro leaves have significant chelating properties, binding to heavy metals in the tissues and helping to carry them outside of the body. Cilantro can be taken as an herbal extract, a tea or consumed regularly in foods as a fresh green.

PECTIN: Pectin is a form of soluble fiber that is found in many fruits, including apples, pears and citrus. In a clinical trial published in "Alternative Therapies in Health and Medicine" in 2008, children with high levels were given pectin supplements to test the detoxification properties of the fiber. Children given pectin had significantly lower levels of lead in the blood, and the excretion of lead through the urine increased by up to 132 percent. Eating pectin-rich fruits in the diet helps with digestion and liver health, supporting proper detoxification by binding toxins and heavy metals, and carrying them out of the body.

MILK THISTLE SEEDS: Milk thistle seeds are used in Western herbal medicine as a protective and toning plant for the liver. In a study published in "The Journal of Biological Research" in 2000, researchers tested the effects of both garlic and milk thistle seeds on animals poisoned with high doses of mercury. In the animals treated with milk thistle seeds, the liver organs were protected against some of the harmful effects of the mercury. Taking milk thistle seeds as a supplement or a herbal tea helps to prevent heavy metal toxicity and supports the functional health of the liver.

GARLIC: According to research, garlic aids in the detoxification of heavy metals. Researchers administered garlic to animals poisoned with heavy metals such as mercury and cadmium. Garlic protected organs from heavy metal toxicity with comparable efficacy to standard prescription drugs and aided in the excretion of cadmium through the feces and urine. Crushed garlic should be consumed fresh, uncooked to preserve its medicinal actions, or it can be taken as a dietary supplement.

CUCUMBER: It is water dense therefore, it is great for eliminating toxins, and it helps dissolve kidney stones and it cleanses and purifies the skin too.

CELERY: It is a natural diuretic so make sure when it is juiced, everything is put into the juicer - stalks and leaves included.

LETTUCE: Lettuce is a natural body cleansers and is dense in nutrients.

CARROTS: It stimulates digestion, cleanses the liver and has a high amount of beta carotene.

CABBAGE: This vegetable is often used and recommended for weight loss, improves poor skin and helps alleviate constipation.

BEETROOT: It is one of the most powerful cleansing foods. It helps cleanse the kidneys, and it even has properties to cleanse the blood.

ASPARAGUS: Asparagus cleanses body tissues and reduces blood acidity.

SPINACH: It is also rich in chlorophyll and helps rebuild the digestive track; stimulates the liver and gall bladder too.

WATERCRESS: A powerful cleanser of the intestines and neutralizes toxins as well. It also helps stimulate fat burning activity. Watercress is good for the skin as well.

APPLES: Apples help control blood pressure, blood sugar levels and helps eliminate body toxins.

Here is a recipe you can enjoy while detoxifying the body:

INGREDIENTS:

1 cucumber

1 large cup of spinach

1 large cup of parsley

1 celery stick

1/2 medium lemon (but not including the peels this time)

INSTRUCTIONS:

Put everything in a juicer and blind. You will be delighted not only with the taste, but also the it detoxify your body.

Detoxifying your body and having a healthier lifestyle does not re☐uire a lot of time or money. You can use simple, healthy ingredients in a moderately priced juicer and get great results.

<u>Chapter 6</u>

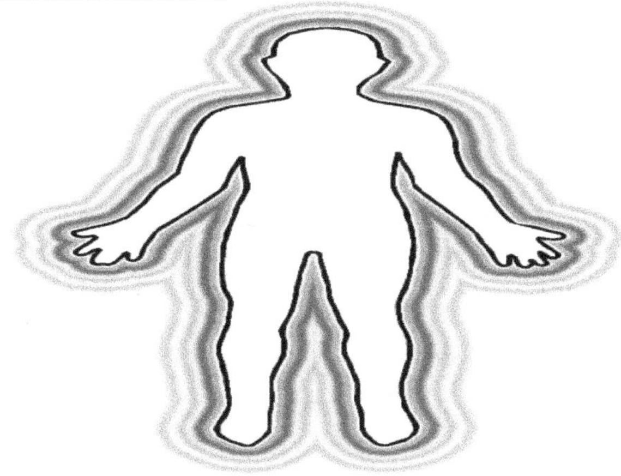

BENEFITS TO DETOXING YOUR BODY AND MIND

There are numerous benefits to effective detoxing that not only occur physically, but also mentally, emotionally, and spiritually. Most of us have heard that by eliminating toxins stored in the body we can experience greater energy, strengthen our immune system, and facilitate healing. Also, when we detox our bodies we can disengage from our habitual thoughts and behaviors and connect more fully with our Inner Being. By freeing ourselves from our toxic habits physically and mentally, we begin to create more wellness throughout our lives.

On a physical level, our bodies are always working to detox, but with the increased factors of internal and external pollution it is difficult for them to keep up. This is especially true when you take into account the diets of most Americans which include refined and processed foods that contribute to a highly acidic diet. Other sources like polluted air, water, electromagnetic fields, and prescription drugs also lead to the toxicity.

By engaging in a detox plan our bodies begin eliminating the toxins that have been accumulated so we can experience greater health and wellness. By the time you have completed an effective detox you will experience increased energy, and an overall feeling of better health. You will notice addictions to sugar and processed foods diminish, while a desire for healthy foods increases.

Detoxing will "reset" your body to a healthier lifestyle, but unless you acqknowledge your cravings for unhealthy foods are gone, you will eventually begin engaging in old unhealthy habits again. Many of us have used food as emotional comfort even if we are unaware of it. By reducing or eliminating our food intake in the form of a detox program we can see what our mental and emotional habits are, and how they affect us.

When doing your fast body detox treatment, pay attention to your thoughts about food. When do you notice cravings arise? Is it your mind or body that is really hungry? Do you use food as a distraction? Often times it is our mind searching for something out of habit, not our body. Pay attention to emotions that arise during your detox, and let go of patterns that are no longer good for you.

THE BASICS OF DETOXING

Depending on what your current health habits are, you will need to choose the best detoxing plan for you. This may range from a specific diet with supplements to a pure fast. Please consult a professional for assistance.   Here are some physical components to consider:

1. Drink plenty of water. Your body will be releasing toxins as you cleanse, and it is important you drink plenty of water to aid in the elimination of these toxins. Drink at least 10-12 eight ounce glasses of water per day, between meals.

2. Drink detox herbal teas to assist the kidneys.

3. Use organic fruits and vegetables if you are eating or juicing.

4. Eat fruits alone. They need their own digestive enzymes and no other food should be eaten for at least 2-3 hours before or after.

5. Use colonics or natural laxative processes (like a saltwater flush) to ensure toxins are being effectively excreted.

6. Eliminate meat and dairy during detox.

7. Reduce or eliminate grains because most are acidic and during a cleanse you want to alkalize your body. (Millet is the exception because it is alkaline.)

8. Move your body. Include light exercise like stretching, yoga, Tai Chi and Chi Gung to help facilitate the movement of toxins. (Avoid strenuous exercise that will produce lactic acid).

9. Take Epsom salt baths to assist the skin with detox.

10. Include deep breathing exercises to help cleanse the lungs.

MENTAL AND EMOTIONAL COMPONENTS:

1. Turn off the TV and eliminate your exposure to the media during your detox. This is a time to go within yourself so be sure to take ☐uiet time for yourself.

2. Journal about the thoughts and feelings you notice during detox, and what you are ready to let go

3. Forgiveness can be a profound aspect of detoxing. Ask yourself who you need to forgive and release it now.

4. Take time each day to recognize what you are grateful for.

Chapter 7

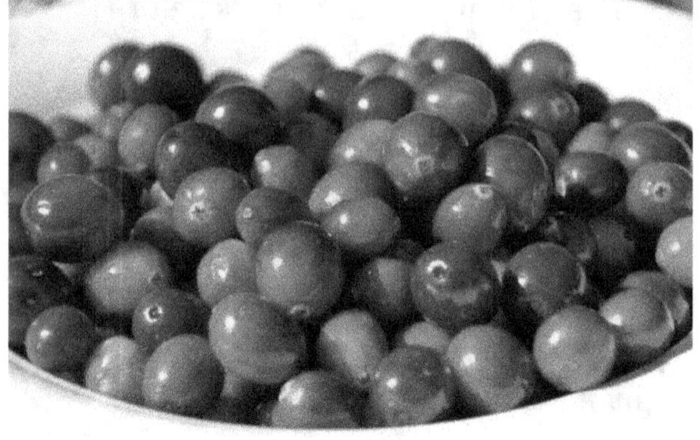

USING CRANBERRYS TO ELLIMINATE TOXICITY IN YOUR BODY

The body accumulates toxins over time from the foods we eat, what we drink, the air we breathe, and chemicals and pollutants in the air. Detox and cleansing diets are often marketed to help rid the body of these toxins and waste products. However, extreme dieting may lead to adverse health concerns. There are a number of healthy foods, including cranberries that can be added to your diet to aid in toxin removal. These berries help eliminate and prevent bacterial growth in the body, and should be part of a well-balanced diet.

ESSENTIAL VITAMINS AND MINERALS

Cranberries are a rich source of essential vitamins and minerals needed for good health. Vitamins and minerals aid in normal body functioning, energy metabolism, and preventing health risks such as heart disease, and stroke. Cranberries are high in vitamins A, B1, B2, B3, B5, B6, and C as well as magnesium, calcium, phosphorus, iron, folic acid, potassium, sodium, and selenium. Many of these nutrients are necessary for healthy liver function to help keep your body in balance.

HEALS THE LIVER

Cranberries help eliminate toxins from the body by detoxing the liver. The liver, which is the largest internal organ in your body, works to support digestion and break down foods that enter your body. Healthy liver function is essential to flushing toxins from the body, as the liver must distinguish between nutrients that need to be absorbed in the body, and toxins that must be eliminated from the blood. The high antioxidant levels of cranberries assist the liver in its detoxification processes.

CRANBERRY JUICE

Cranberry juice aids the body in flushing out harmful toxins. The juice has antibacterial properties that inhibit bacterial overgrowth in the body that contribute to poor digestion or urinary tract infections. Increased bacteria in the body leads to toxin accumulation and increased health risks. Cranberry juice works to cleanse the lymphatic system that works to neutralize waste products to eliminate toxins from the body's tissues. Be aware of commercially prepared juices that are sold in most supermarkets. Many of these juices have added sugars or other juices such as apple or grape juices. Look for a brand that is labeled unsweetened and mix juices with filtered water to decrease natural sweetness or calories.

WELL-BALANCED DIET

There is no one magical food that will help detoxify the body to eliminate toxins. Rather, it is essential to eat a well-balanced diet that contains essential nutrients, vitamins and minerals. In addition to adding cranberries to your diet, be sure to eat a variety of fruits and vegetables, complex carbohydrates, lean proteins and healthy fats. When possible, purchase organic produce and meats that are free from hormones, antibiotics or pesticides to decrease toxicity in your body. Add cranberries to your daily diet plan by drinking cranberry juice with your breakfast, as a snack, adding cranberries to a milk smoothie or a bowl of oatmeal for a healthy antioxidant boost.

Chapter 8

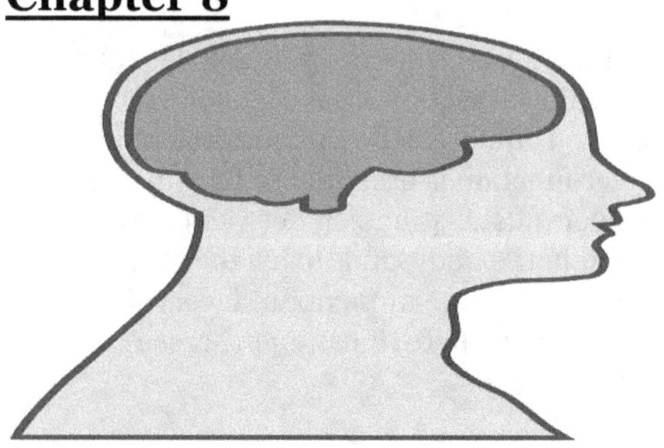

HOW DETOXIFICATION WILL IMPROVE YOUR MENTAL HEALTH

Detoxification refers to a cleansing or purification process. It involves the transformation and elimination of bodily waste: Toxins that impair physical organ function, and affect mental well-being and cognitive function.

Trauma is toxic beyond the metaphor often used to describe "toxic relationships; stress creates inflammation and metabolic byproducts that cannot be as easily eliminated.

Many people are exposed to chemical and biological toxins in the course of trauma, for example, war, natural disasters, and genocide or have used toxic substances such as alcohol. These toxins affect all aspect of physical and mental health including brain function.

Poor ☐uality nutrition also contributes to the buildup of toxins in the body as a natural by-product of daily life which suggests everyone can benefit from engaging in detoxification strategies. Everyone can benefit from activities that support detoxification.

Detoxification is an essential part of a prevention and treatment program for recovery of mental health, including PTSD, depression, and addictions. Every culture includes a variety of detoxification methods in their traditional medicine repertoire.

The Liver is the Major Detox Organ

The liver and the skin are the major organs of detoxification in the body. The liver is the human body's largest organ, and a primary organ of detoxification.

Whether one is detoxifying from pharmaceuticals, drugs or alcohol, or undertaking detoxification strategies to enhance health, the process is similar.

The Liver is the center for detoxification in the body and undergoes two interrelated processes, phase 1 and phase 2 detoxification. During phase 1, the liver makes fat-soluble toxins water-soluble by activating the Cytochrome P-450 enzymes. These enzymes attach to toxins and prepare them for phase 2 detoxification, where they are then eliminated by the kidneys. Symptoms of liver and gall bladder congestion include nausea, morning headaches, bloodshot eyes, skin problems, constipation, light colored or poorly formed stools, pain in the upper shoulders or under the rib cage.

Plants That Help the Liver Detox

Many Indigenous societies use alterative (blood-purifying) plants like Burdock to detoxify. Bitter plants that stimulate digestion like, dandelion and bitter root (Lewisia rediviva) are prized by Pacific Northwest natives for their cleansing properties. Purslane (Portulaca oleracea), also called verdolaga in Mexico is eaten to enhance digestion and stimulate the liver's work. Japanese people use charcoal made from bamboo to purify spaces; activated charcoal remains the treatment for accidental poisoning (this should be used only under professional guidance) in humans and animals. Fibers, and barks are also used to absorb and eliminate toxins as well as soothe the sensitive lining of the stomach and intestines like the nutritious slippery elm bark (Ulmas rubra).

Foods that Help the Liver Detox and aid in Alcohol Recovery

Foods are important as both a cause of toxins and in supporting the elimination of toxins. The cruciferous vegetables like cabbage, broccoli, and Brussels sprouts enhance the liver's P-450 enzymes, and sulphur-containing onions and garlic, both raw and cooked, should be used daily.

Bread and yeast based products can cause toxicity especially for those sensitive to alcohol. Yeast ferments sugar into alcohol and endogenous alcohol production is high after eating foods rich in carbohydrates). Yeasts convert the alcohol (ethanol) into acetaldehyde affecting levels of gut flora and leading to chronic candidiasis. The acetaldehyde toxins can also cause leaky gut which is implicated in allergies and autoimmune illnesses.

SEAWEEDS: Seaweed is one of the most important detoxifying foods because they bind toxins in the intestinal tract. Adding seaweed to soups or bean dishes or as a snack is healthy for the thyroid, and also as part of detoxifying. Alginates from the brown seaweeds bind toxic metals and radioactive isotopes in the digestive tract.

Seaweed Detox Recipe

This salad uses hijike or arame sea vegetables, which are among the mildest seaweeds. This salad is a good first step in exploring seaweeds in recipes. It is especially beneficial for fatigue, depression, and hypothyroidism.

1 cup of dry arame or hijiki seaweed

3 scallions

1 cup tofu

1 carrot

½ cup peapods

½ of a red bell pepper

½ of an English cucumber

Handful of broccoli florets

¼ cup walnuts or pine nuts

Sprouts (optional)

Dressing

¼ cup toasted sesame oil

¼ cup rice wine vinegar

1 tablespoon wheat-free tamari

Juice from of 2 cloves of garlic and a chunk of fresh ginger

Dash of hot red pepper flakes (optional)

Directions

1.   Soak the seaweed in warm water for 15 minutes until soft (save the water for soup or to put in your animal companion's bowl).

2.   Dice the scallions, tofu, carrots, peapods, red pepper, cucumber, broccoli, nuts, and sprouts (if using) into small (eＱual size) pieces.

3.   Mix all of the dressing ingredients together in a bowl and whisk until well combined.

4. Combine the vegetable mixture with the softened seaweed and pour the dressing over it. Mix and allow to marinate for a few hours. Eat and enjoy!

Purge-and-cleanse systems that detox

Purge-and-cleanse systems traditionally include the use of clays, plant and animal-derived oils, sweat lodges, saunas, water therapies, induced-regurgitation, and enemas to detoxify the body and reestablish metabolic balance. The use of sweats and enemas and cleansing teas are found throughout the world cultures.

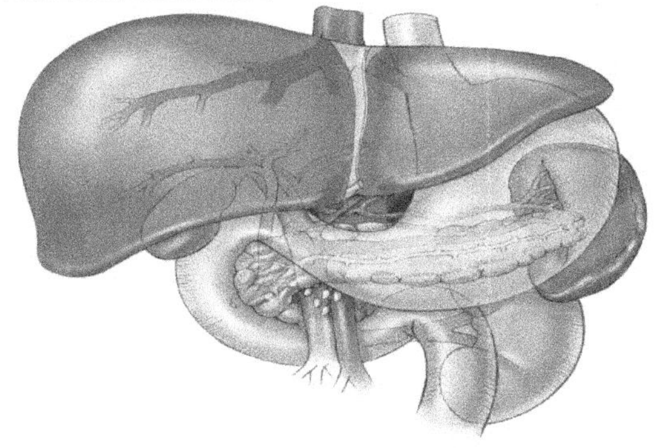

Chapter 9

HOW TO CLEANSE THE LIVER OF TOXINS

The liver is the largest internal organ in your body. It is a very complex, vital organ that has many functions. Some include breaking down fats from the foods you consume and filtering out disease-causing toxins from your bloodstream. Every day your body is continuously exposed to harmful toxins such as medications, environmental pollutants and artificial chemicals in foods. Your liver depends on you to take care of it. Luckily, there are many ways you can detoxify your liver and make it effective in eliminating harmful toxins.

Step 1

Take a 500 mg vitamin C (ascorbic acid) capsule. These should be taken once a day. Vitamin C helps detoxify your liver. This vitamin aids your liver in making glutathione, an antioxidant that helps the liver flush out toxins. Additionally, eat two to three servings of healthy foods high in vitamin C every day along with your supplements. Foods rich in vitamin C include all citrus fruits, green and red peppers, tomatoes, berries, and broccoli.

Step 2

Consume two to three servings of healthy foods rich in fiber. Your liver brings the toxins that enter your body straight to your digestive system. When your digestive system has enough fiber, the toxins bind with the food that you eat are eliminated with your next bowel movement. When your digestive system doesn't have enough fiber, the toxins are circulated back into your blood and your liver becomes overworked because it has to process them all over again. Foods high in fiber include wheat bread, whole grains, flaxseeds, corn, prunes, apples, beans, and pineapples.

Step 3

Drink water. Consume 10 to 12 glasses of water daily. Drinking enough water will help your liver flush out toxins. Drink filtered or bottled water to avoid taking in bad elements in tap water or public drinking fountains.

Step 4

Exercise for one hour. Exercising for an hour every day will help stimulate your liver and other internal organs. Exercises such as aerobics, jogging, running, and strength training will stimulate your liver to flush out toxins while improving your blood circulation and cardiovascular health. Consult your doctor before embarking on any kind of exercise routine.

WARNINGS

The Secrets of Body Toxins and Detox Preparation With the Real Deal Fitness and Wellness System

For thousands of years every major culture and religion has emphasised the importance of cleansing the body through fasting and/or special diets to rest the body, and enable it to heal itself. The body detox is not a new idea, but a proven method of helping you to feel and look fantastic!

We live in a world polluted by substances that create an irritating or harmful effect in the body. These substances are known as toxins. They can interfere with the normal body functions, and are absorbed into the body externally (e.g.

through the skin, inhaled or eaten) or internally (as a by-product of normal bodily processes). We have never been more exposed to toxins because of our polluted environment and processed food diets. Therefore the need to help the body cleanse and heal itself has never been greater.

Some of the external toxins that we are exposed to come from:

> Car and industrial plant fumes, tobacco smoke.

> Tap water containing heavy metals, industrial/agricultural chemicals and chlorine (absorbed through drinking and the skin when taking a bath or shower).

> Pesticides, herbicides, preservatives, synthetic additives, antibiotics and growth hormones (in meat) in the processed non-organic food we eat.

> Household air fresheners and cleaners, skin creams, deodorants, shampoos, hairsprays, damp proof and furniture treatments and electromagnetic pollution from home electronic gadgets.

At the same time our bodies continually produce toxins from all the processes that are needed to keep us alive, such as breathing, digestion, and immunity system defence. Sources of internal toxins include:

> Free radicals (unstable molecules) generated from normal body processes that can cause havoc in the body (e.g. they have been linked to ageing and cancer).

> The by-products of bacteria and yeasts that live in our intestines.

> Injuries and wounds.

> Excessive stress.

> Mercury or "silver" tooth fillings.

If the rate at which toxins are absorbed or created exceeds the rate of removal then they accumulate in different parts of the body. As more toxins accumulate symptoms of toxicity start to show, and more fat is created to store them. This situation develops much faster if you lack enough sleep, have a negative attitude, eat a lot of products containing sugar, smoke, drink more alcohol than recommended guidelines, and lead a stressful lifestyle.

There are many possible symptoms, but some of the common ones include unaccountable aches and pains in the joints, allergies, skin rashes and spots, backache, bad breath/body odour, depression, fre☐uent mood swings, poor concentration, lack of energy, nausea, furred tongue, regular headaches/migraines, strong smelling urine, and susceptibility to colds and infections. There are a range of subjective ☐uestions that you can use to estimate how toxic you are.

A detox is simply a way to help the body to get rid of the toxins so that it can begin healing itself. It will leave you feeling more alert, with more energy, able to breathe easier, your skin will be clearer, you will feel happier, and more able to deal with life in general. Irritating health problems (e.g. allergies, skin rashes) may completely disappear, and you will suddenly remember what it is like to be healthy again!

You can support the body systems that remove toxins by eating more of certain foods. Some of the organs that are involved in filtering and clearing toxins from your body include the liver, spleen, gall bladder, and gastro-intestinal tract. There are a variety of natural foods and supplements that can support these organs and help them to function better. These include Asparagus, Broccoli, Brussels sprouts, Cabbage, Carrots, Cauliflower, Garlic, Onions, Peppers, Seeds (e.g. flax, sunflower and pumpkin), Tomatoes, Watercress, Lemons, Pineapple, Dandelion, Fennel, Ginger, Nettle, Cayenne pepper, Cinnamon, and Ginseng.

Another body system involved in removing toxins is the immune system. This includes the spleen, white blood cells, the tonsils, thymus and lymphatic system. Some of the natural foods and supplements that can support these organs include Artichoke, Basil, Sprouted seeds, Chives, Cinnamon, Mint, Thyme, Cloves, Cucumber, Cumin, Green beans, Pulses, Unrefined cereals, Apples, Blackberries, Cherries, Raspberries, Echinacea, Li☐uorice root and Olive leaf.

All airborne toxins are dealt with by the respiratory system, from the mucous membranes and hair in your nose to the lungs. Foods and supplements to support this system include Basil, Chives and lettuce, Marjoram, Parsley, Radish, Rosemary, Thyme and Mullein.

The primary function of the kidneys and urinary system is to filter out toxins from the blood and eliminate them through the urine. The urinary tract consists of the urethras (the tubes that drain the kidneys), the bladder and the urethra (the tube that empties the bladder). Foods and supplements that help this system include Barley, Celery, Leek, and Wheat germ, Blackcurrant, Blueberry, Fig, Horsetail, and Goldenrod.

The largest organ in the body and our primary defensive shell against our polluted environment is the skin. One of its functions is to remove toxins through sweating. This is why saunas are traditionally used to detox. Skin health is supported for example, red/green/yellow fruit/vegetables, Cabbage, Carrots, Flax and Pumpkin seeds, Camomile, Gingko Biloba, and Evening Primrose oil.

During and after a detox there will always be some side effects. The strength of these will depend on your level of toxicity and the strength of the detox you choose to use. There are many ways to vary the strength by changing the length of the detox, what you eat (fasting is the strongest form), and taking detox supplements. The side effects may be uncomfortable in the short term, but when you feel the benefits afterwards it will be well worth it!

In the week before the detox there are a few things that you can do to make it enjoyable and less stressful. Mental preparation includes setting aside the time for your detox as a break from all of your normal routines and making sure that you have a clear idea of your motivation to detox. It is important for you and your family to be prepared for an emotional rollercoaster of mixed feelings, caused by the detox. If possible, you may want to arrange to be alone for the first few days of a strong detox, and in any case be prepared for family and friends scepticism. Just remember that when they see the results they will want to detox too!

In terms of physical preparation you may want to consider the following:

> Pamper yourself with massage, steam treatments and saunas.

> Reduce your intake of addictive substances such as nicotine, caffeine, chocolate, sugar and alcohol.

> Alter your diet to reduce your intake of meat, fish, and dairy products.

> As special treats during the detox, buy some good reading material and/or films, aromatherapy candles, lavender oil, and essential oils for the bath.

> Finally there will be a list of special foods, drinks, and supplements to be bought for the detox.

Conclusion

Thank you again for downloading this book!

I hope this book was able to help you to understand the importance of keeping your body and mind free of all toxins.

A body toxin may be defined as any substance that is potentially injurious, destructive, or fatal to human health. Some toxins come from dietary or environmental sources, some are manufactured within the body, and all toxins are potentially harmful because they are part of the process of developing illness and disease.

The human body contains a natural detoxifying system. Normally, toxins are processed through the liver, kidneys, and lower intestines. These organs convert toxins to a more benign substance or they eliminate them out of the body in order to prevent damage to other, more delicate organs like the heart and stomach. However, the natural process of detoxification is not always able to handle the amount of toxins that are introduced into the body through the diet and the environment. Sometimes additional attention, and help, is needed to reduce the introduction of toxins into the body, and to remove unwanted toxins already in the body.

If your diet includes a high level of fat or sugar, coffee or alcohol, smoke cigarettes, take any drugs or medications, or are exposed to harmful environmental chemicals from any source, you may want to consider detoxing your body. Symptoms that indicate an accumulation of toxins include fatigue, irritability, skin problems, digestive difficulties, aches and pains, and constipation. Sometimes these symptoms can indicate a more serious medical problem so it may be a good idea to consult with your doctor.

Many people have found that dietary changes, colon cleanses, saunas, or taking vitamins, herbs and other supplements can be effective ways to detoxify the body. Most detoxification programs include drinking lots of water or juice. Drinking herbal teas is another cost-effective way to aid in purifying the body. Many herbs contain powerful antioxidants, which are substances that protect against cell damage.

Detoxification will improve immune functions, purify blood, and reduce the amount of toxins in the body that will reduce the burden on the body's organs. People who have gone through a detoxification process have noticed many benefits. A few of these include: Improved energy, stress relief, improved skin health, reduced headaches, and other aches and pains.

To begin your detox program, make sure you do your research, and find a time-proven detox program that is gentle on the body's system. Try to talk to other people who have gone through the detox program, and hear what their experience was, and what benefits they have gained.

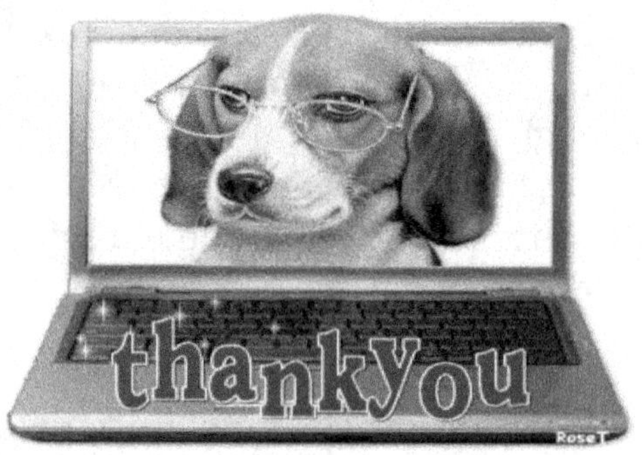

Finally, if you enjoyed this book, then I'd like to ask you for a favor, would you be kind enough to leave a review for this book on Amazon? It'd be greatly appreciated!

Thank you and good luck!

Chapter 1

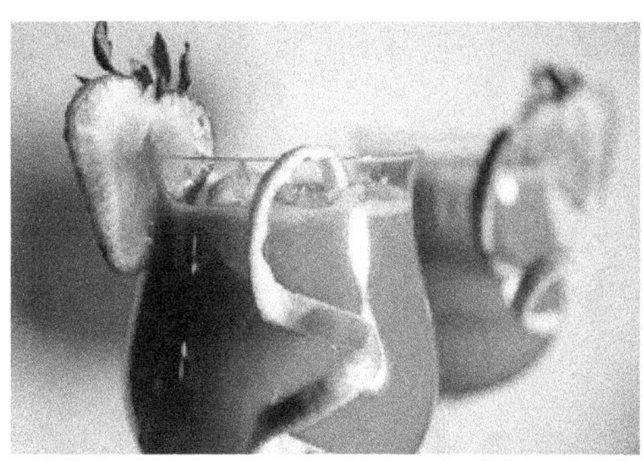

Berry A-Peeling

Ingredients

Apples-2 large (3-1/4" dia)

Lime-1/2 fruit (2" dia)

Strawberries-3 cup, whole

Directions: Process all ingredients in a juicer, shaker or stir and serve

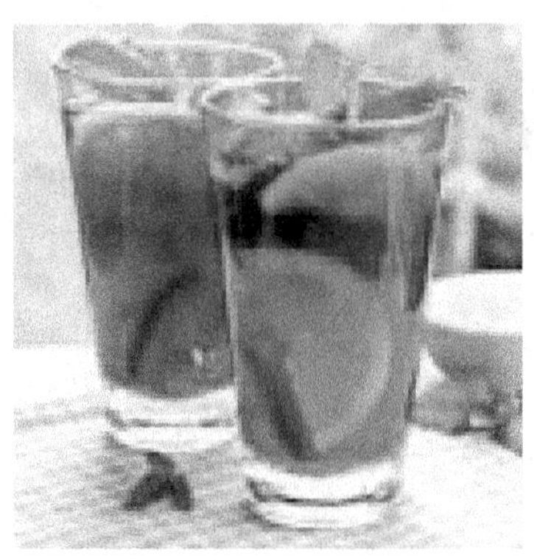

Minty Berry

Ingredients

Blueberries-2 cup

Kiwifruit-2 fruit (2"dia)

Peppermint-30 leaves

Strawberry-1 cup, whole

Directions: Process all ingredients in a juicer, shaker or stir and serve

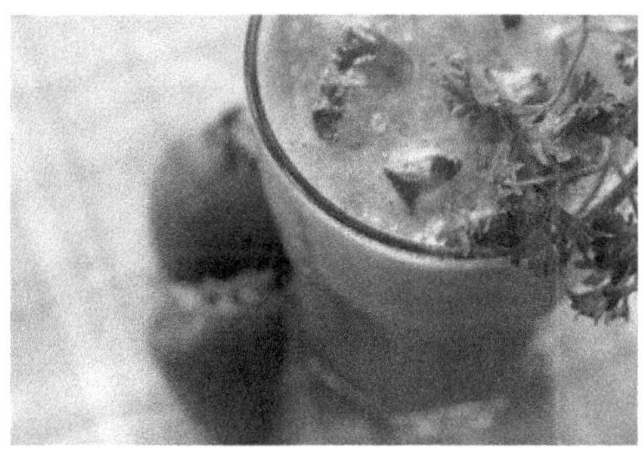

Red Dawn

Ingredients

Apples-2 medium (3" dia)

Cabbage (red)-2 leaf

Carrots-3 medium

Cucumber-1 cucumber (8-1/4")

Mango (peeled)-1 fruit without refuse

Strawberries-1.5 cup, whole

Directions: Process all ingredients in a juicer, shaker or stir and serve

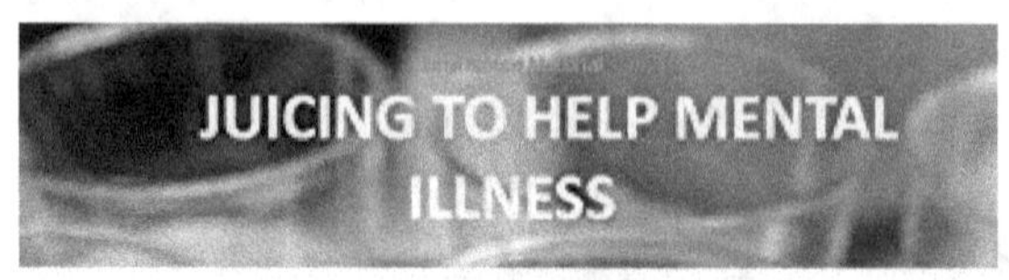

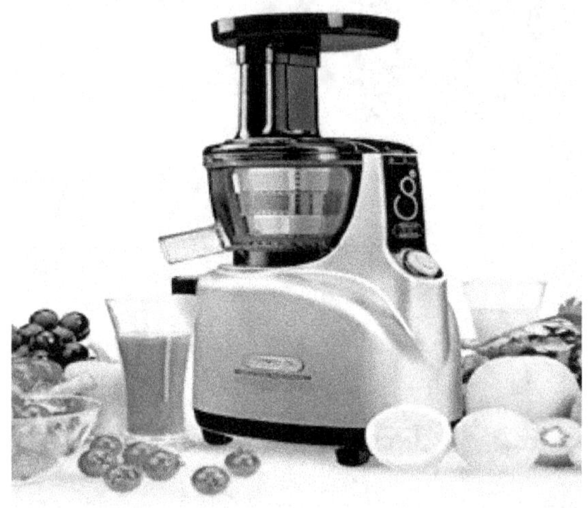

To check out the rest of (JUICING TO HELP MENTAL ILLNESS: Awesome Juicing Recipes For A Healthier Mental Health Experience) go to Amazon.com

Check Out My Other Books

Below you'll find some of my other popular books that are popular on Amazon and Kindle as well.   Alternatively, you can visit my author page on Amazon to see other work done by me.

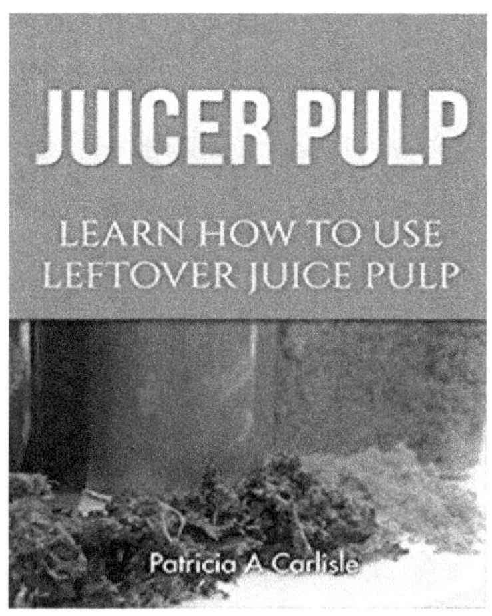

JUICER PULP: LEARN HOW TO USE LEFTOVER JUICE PULP.

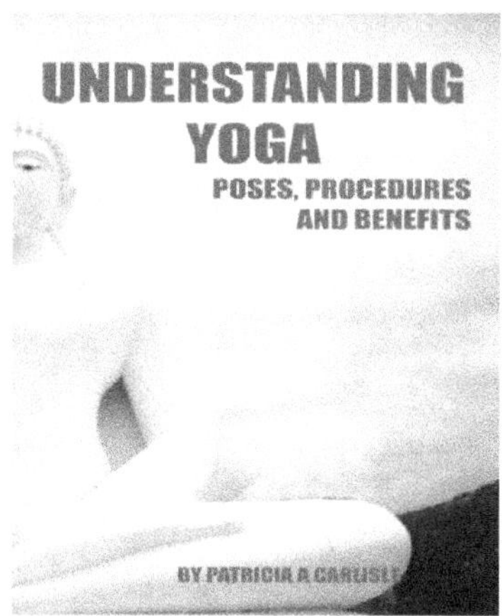

UNDERSTANDING YOGA: POSES, PROCEDURES AND BENEFITS.

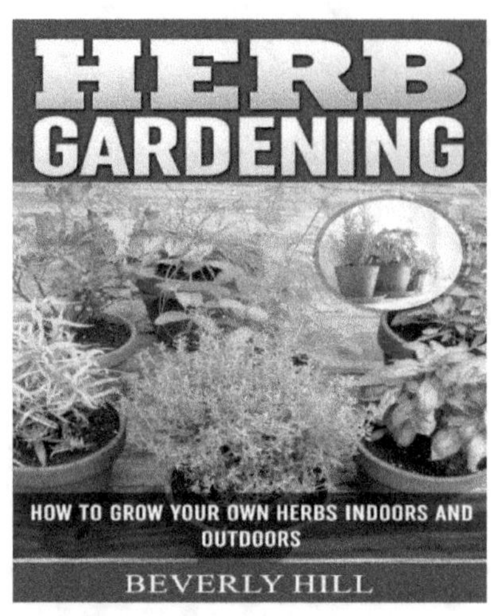

HERB GARDENING: HOW TO GROW YOUR OWN HERBS INDOORS AND OUTDOORS.

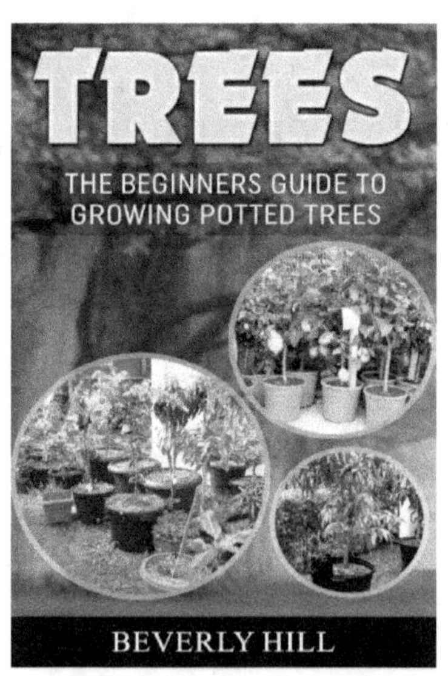

TREES: THE BEGINNERS GUIDE TO GROWING POTTED TREES.

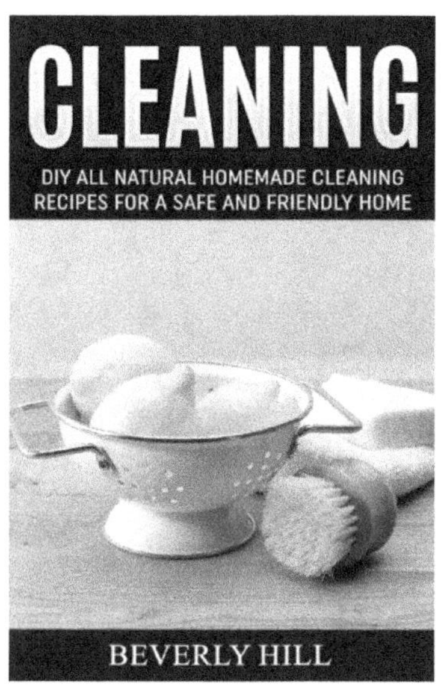

CLEANING: DIY ALL NATURAL HOMEMADE CLEANING RECIPES FOR A SAFE AND FRIENDLY HOME.

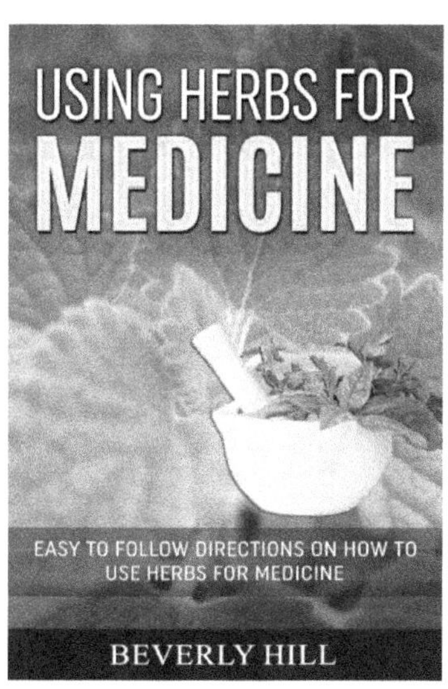

USING HERBS FOR MEDICINE: EASY TO FOLLOW DIRECTIONS ON HOW TO USE HERBS FOR MEDICINE.

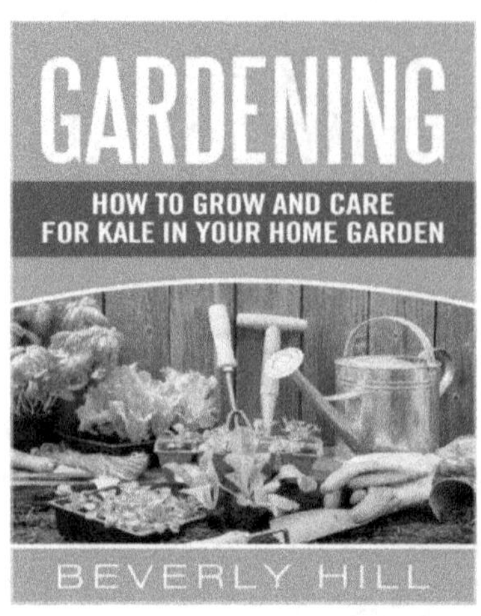

GARDENING: HOW TO GROW AND CARE FOR KALE IN YOUR HOME GARDEN.

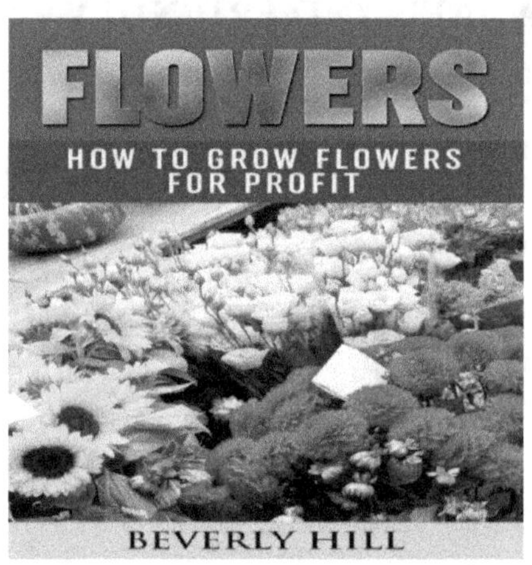

FLOWERS: HOW TO GROW FLOWERS FOR PROFIT.

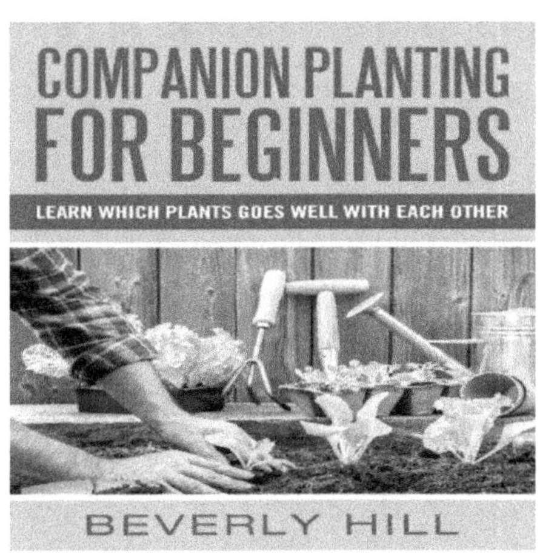

COMPANIOR PLANTING FOR BEGINNERS: LEARN WHICH PLANTS WORKS WILL WITH EACH OTHER.

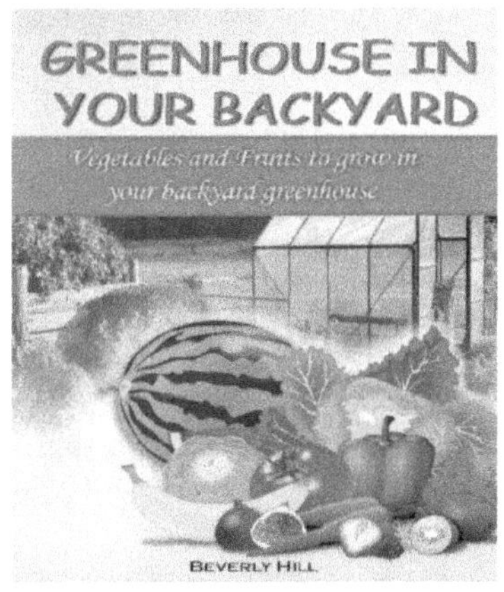

GREENHOUSE IN YOUR BACKYARD: VEGETABLES AND FRUITS TO GROW IN YOUR BACKYARD GREENHOUSE:

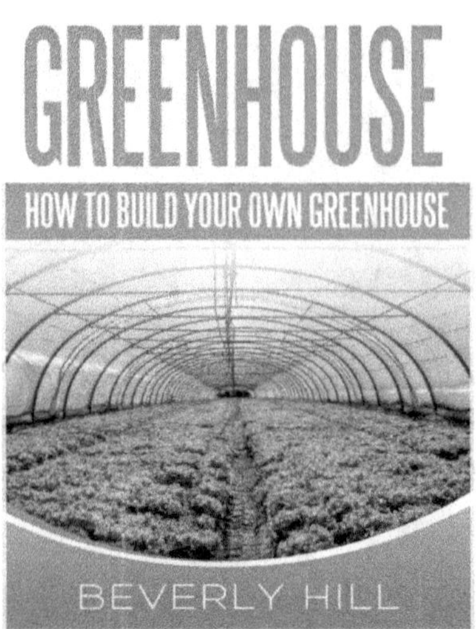

GREENHOUSE: HOW TO BUILD YOUR OWN GREENHOUSE.

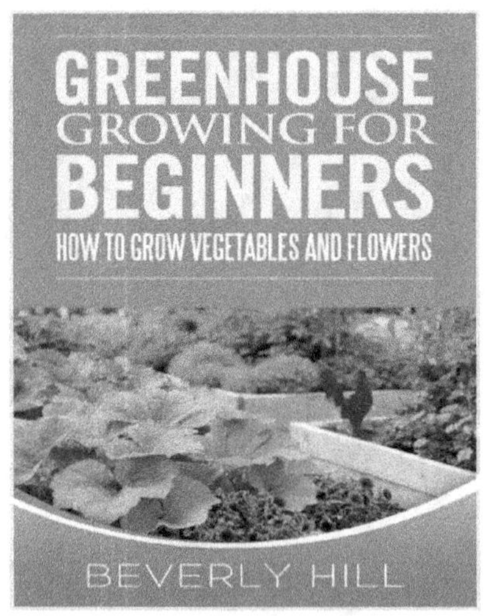

GREENHOUSE GROWING FOR BEGINNERS: HOW TO GROW VEGETABLES AND FLOWERS.

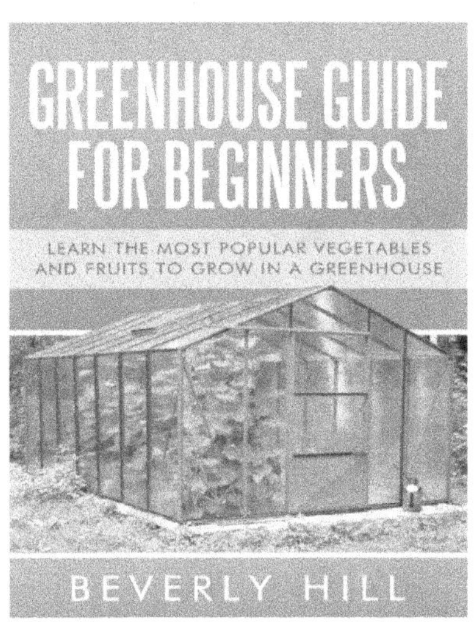

GREENHOUSE GUIDE FOR BEGINNERS: LEARN THE MOST POPULAR VEGETABLES AND FRUITS TO GROW IN A GREENHOUSE.

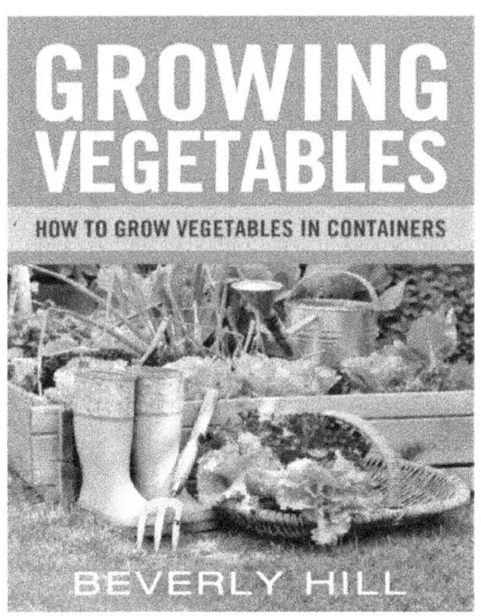

GROWING VEGETABLES: HOW TO GROW VEGETABLES IN CONTAINERS.

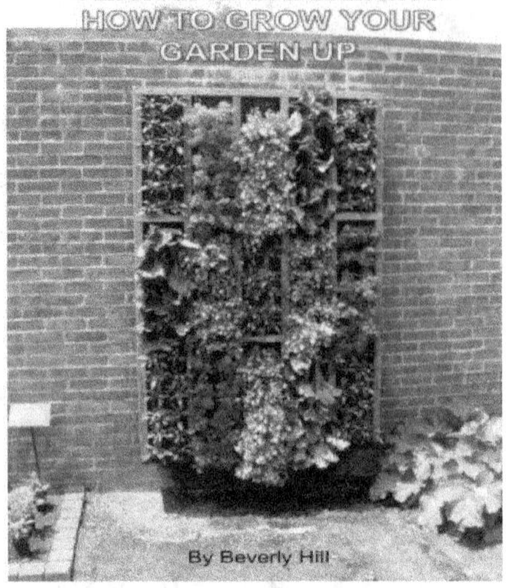

VERTICAL GARDENING: HOW TO GROW YOUR GARDEN UP.

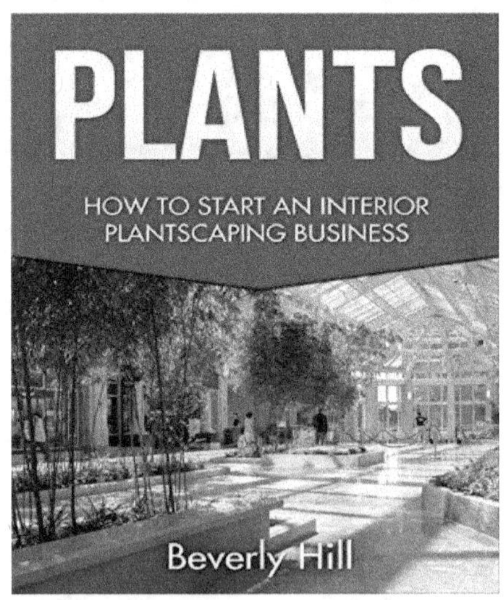

PLANTS: HOW TO START AN INTERIOR PLANTSCAPING BUSINESS.

BONUS: SUBSCRIBE TO THE FREE BOOK

Beginners Guide to Yoga & Meditation

"Stressed out? Do You Feel Like The World Is Crashing Down Around You? Want To Take A Vacation That Will Relax Your Mind, Body And Spirit? Well this Easy To Read Step By Step

E-Book Makes It All Possible!"

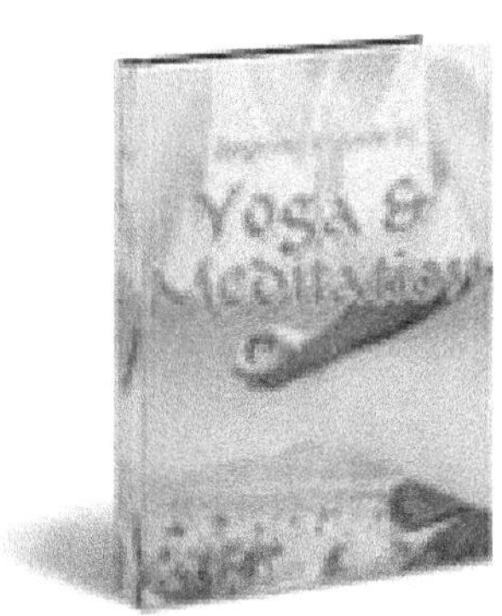

Instructions on how to join our mailing list, and receive a free copy of "Yoga and Meditation" can be found in any of my Kindle eBooks.

NOTES

NOTES

NOTES

NOTES